From The Author to the Reader

E very day is a brand new opportunity! We must seize the day - seize the opportunity and make it a habit to be in the mode of "Always Learning!"

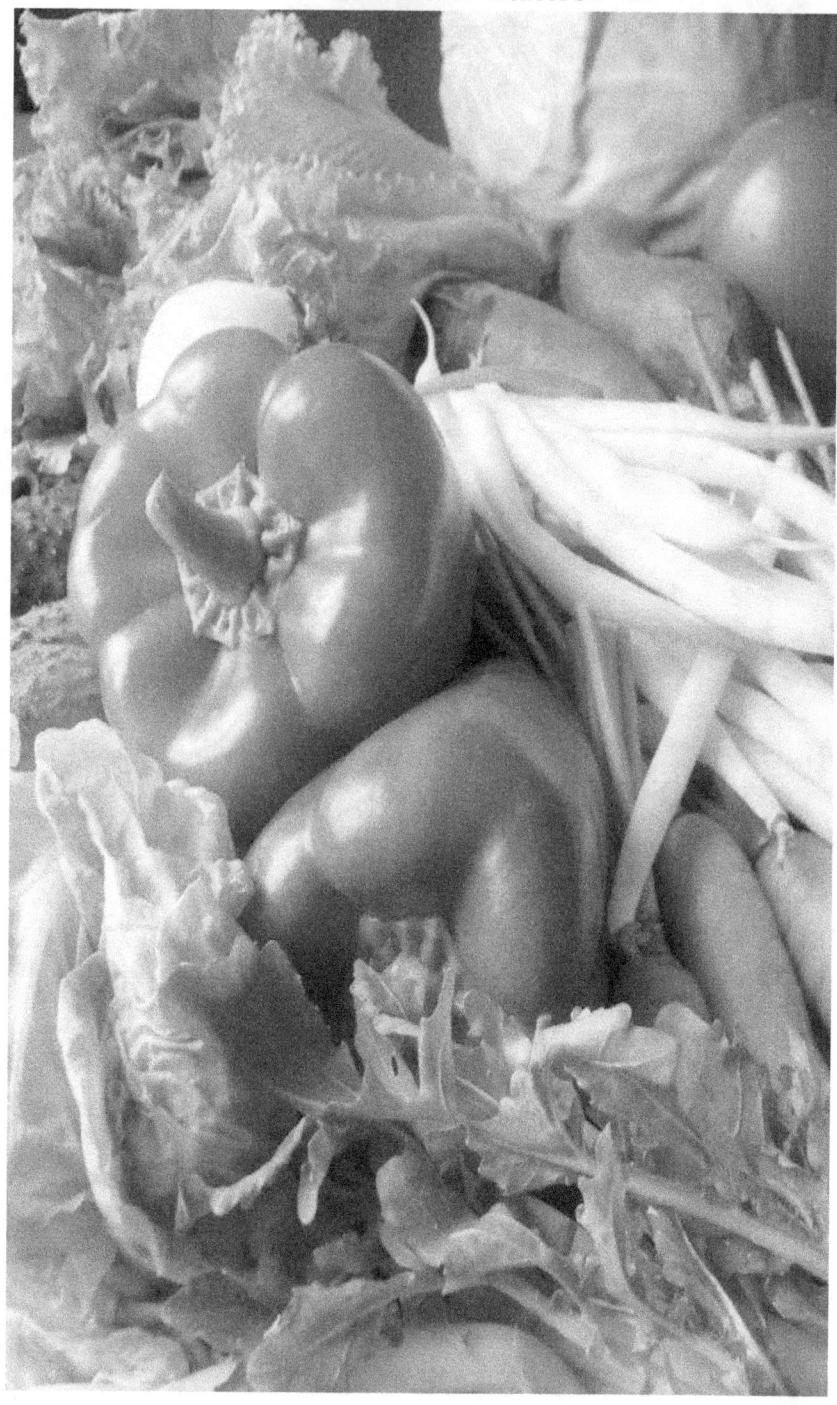

Apple Cider Vinegar Benefits

Barbara B Walters

Apple Cider Vinegar Benefits

Top Secret Detox Recipes, Health and Beauty Remedies and Cures

To Cleanse and Detox for Faster Weight Loss

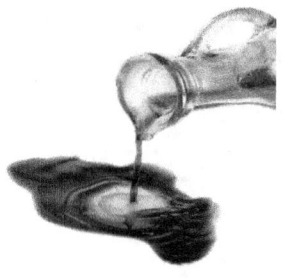

Barbara B Walters

Copyright Notice and Disclaimer

First Printing, 2014

ISBN-13: 978-1495480423

DEDICATION

To Betsy and Tobias, Lewis,
Charles and Debbie

Contents

Preface

Apple Cider Vinegar Miracle Health Elixir

Besides having many oral health benefits, apple cider vinegar is well known to offer a broad variety of topical application functions and lots of beauty usages.

Apple cider vinegar also known as cider vinegar or ACV is a light to amber color vinegar and is made from apple or cider.

It can be used as a bath soak, age spot removal, facial toner, getting rid of acne, hair rinse, facial peel, foot soak, sunburn treatment, deodorant, helps to relieves arthritis pain, clear up nasal congestion and fix broken veins and bruises.

It is simple and very affordable to make good quality all-natural, unfiltered and unpasteurized apple cider vinegar at home. Fermentation time will depend on the approach selected for making it. Whole apples or cores and peels may be used.

It's best to use the scraps, peels and core method because it allows you to enjoy the apple and at the same time make use of the waste to prepare and get the highest quality vinegar.

It will take approximately two months for the apple cider vinegar to ferment from scraps and around six months from whole apples. In addition, there are several other methods to make apple cider vinegar on a large scale for commercial purposes.

For commercial synthesis apples are crushed to squeeze out the juice. Bacteria and yeast may be added to encourage alcoholic fermentation and its process. Sugars present in apples are converted into alcohol during this process.

In the second half of the fermentation process, alcohol gets converted into vinegar by the action of bacteria called acetobacter, which helps in the formation of acetic acid. Malic acid and acetic acid gives vinegar its sour taste.

The primary content of vinegar is acetic acid but it can include other vitamins, acids, minerals, amino acids and fiber.

Even with various case studies of individuals who had remarkable relief with cider vinegar in their daily conditions, the medical establishment often disregarded the claims of cider vinegar out of hand, as they were not part of a scientifically measured trial.

Clearly, we need more scientific research to back up personal experience; however a broad selection of anecdotal sources would indeed suggest that it works.

Still few studies indicate that numerous claims made through experience of generations needed more in depth study to understand and fully utilize the unknown factual health benefits behind its working. Apple cider vinegar has started regaining its popularity as a health tonic and nutritional supplement.

Few research have stated that it is highly effect in healing diabetes, obesity, heart diseases, fighting infections, fighting yeast infection, hypertension, reducing heart burn, helping in digestion, relieving leg cramps, fighting bad breath, boosting metabolism, tiredness, reducing swelling, killing foot fungus and lowering cholesterol levels.

Individuals who consume apple cider vinegar with their meals experience fullness for a longer period of time. It additionally regularizes bowel movement and lowers heart burn. It is also proven to alleviate chest congestion as well as boosts energy.

It works as a blood thinner, provides relief from jelly fish sting, skin irritation, bug bites and helps in lowering blood pressure.

Is It Safe?

Vinegar is safe and edible, and it cannot hurt your stomach when ingested in small quantities. Multiple sorts and flavors of vinegars are available, in regards to food enhancements and vinaigrettes.

The world of culinary vinegars is a big one. Many types of vinegar are flavored by the addition of herbs or fruits; raspberry vinegar is one of the very popular.

For the diet conscious, vinegar is fat free and low in sodium. According to the studies conducted in relation to vinegar and weight loss, it has been concluded that it might reduce body weight and obesity.

More studies are needed to fully understand the working and relationship to weight reduction. Very high intake for a long period of time may lead to hyperreninemia, hyperkalemia and osteoporosis, so proper care and precautions are recommended during the continuous use of ACV.

Apple cider vinegar has been associated with providing natural remedies for many kinds of chronic diseases such as, acid reflux, acne, constipation, weight loss, reduce blood sugar, memory problems, and reversing aging.

Apple cider vinegar also acts as a blood thinner and may also help in the prevention of high blood pressure, as mentioned above from centuries ago, ACV has been considered to be the father of all cures.

During various wars it was used as an antiseptic to treat the wounds. It is known to work as a natural detoxifying agent, providing relief from allergies, balancing the body pH, reducing inflammation and preventing flu.

Apples being highly nutritious fruit contain a wide variety of vitamins, minerals, amino acids, enzymes, pectin, and others. Apples are the core ingredient in apple cider vinegar, so this fluid contains these nutritional benefits as well.

All vinegars do not possess the same kind of natural remedial value as apple cider vinegar does. It also contains many enzymes, microbes, and all the bye products produced during the processing.

Making Your Own Vinegar

You can make your very own apple cider vinegar at home and be comfortable with its quality and purity without having doubts that you might have about the available commercial brands.

Start with a sweet based fluid of your choice as it can be created from anything containing sugar or starch. Cider or aged wine or a different fruit juice is usually the simplest to use.

The top of your container should be covered with cheesecloth, but not air tight as you'll need the bacteria in the air to allow it to ferment. It may look bad but it is good. If your vinegar seems too strong, add a little water.

Once you are happy with the flavor, transfer the liquid into a clean bottle through a paper coffee filter. Seal with a cork (the vinegar will corrode a metal top).

Keep your vinegar in a dark warm place. This is not a quick process. It will take many weeks to several months - or more - to produce vinegar that you will enjoy.

Vinegar can be made from many fruits, vegetables and grains but apple cider vinegar as the name suggests is made from pulverized apples. No other vinegar possesses the same qualities and benefits as ACV.

From being used as a folk remedy it has recently gained a more modern approach on its uses and benefits based on studies and researches. Apple cider vinegar may also be used with medication for diabetes and heart diseases as well as with laxatives and diuretics (speak with your doctor).

Food drug interactions need to be understood fully by patients utilizing these medications for their treatment before starting on a new remedy.

Vinegar also helps in purifying and detoxifying many body organs. It assists in oxidizing of blood, neutralizing toxic body substances and pathogenic bacteria, and promotes the digestion and elimination process.

There are also claims of it helping in the strengthening of the heart and anti-carcinogenic effects on certain types of cancers. Vinegar contains chromium which could have an altering effect on your insulin level.

The Nutrition Benefits
Behind Apple Cider Vinegar

It is often these elements giving vinegar its healthful qualities and nature, although most commercial vinegar these days is filtered to take out the main source "the mother" as well as any sediment.

It's very sad that, lots of people feel vinegar is a superior product as it is more aesthetically appealing, so producers comply by pasteurizing and filtering the vinegar they make. This process stops the activity of the acetobacter bacteria.

The end result is vinegar whose quality may be regulated and assured, but is lacking a number of the critical qualities that makes it so powerful and successful for health benefits. Removing the "mother" and sediments of vinegar also lessens the complexity of flavors in the vinegar.

Like processed flour and pasteurized juices which have had nutrients removed or destroyed, vinegar which is filtered and pasteurized is commercially acceptable, but less successful nutritionally.

Apples are a nutritional powerhouse and truly deserving of the legendary phrase; an apple a day keeps the doctor away. They contain a wide variety of nutrients, such as pectin (soluble fiber), beta-carotene (an antioxidant), and lots of minerals.

Introduction

It is no secret that vegetables and fruits are good for you. You probably already know a few of the health benefits, including lower blood pressure treat diabetes, cardiovascular disease, stroke and certain cancers.

You might even understand that eating fresh fruits and vegetables may lower your chance of losing your eyesight as you get older. Yes, vegetables and fruits are rich in vitamins, a large number of fiber and health protective compounds.

But are you aware that consuming more of these is a vital strategy in **losing weight** and **keeping it off?** With the exception of a few starchy vegetables, a large proportion is quite low in calories.

That's because they're mostly made up of water and fiber (both of which have no calories). Studies show that the more vegetables and fruits people eat, the less they tend to weigh.

It truly can be as easy as eating a salad. In a recent study at Pennsylvania State University, women who consumed a meal with a low-calorie salad and then ate a pasta meal had about 12% less calories than women who started with the pasta and skipped the salad.

With some exceptions, there's absolutely no need to avoid this vegetable or that fruit since it contains sugar or will raise your blood sugar.

Most fruits and veggies are actually very low in total carbs and contain fiber - often the soluble fiber that slows blood sugar's rise - therefore their GLs are quite low. So don't hesitate to snack on apples and pile your plate with vegetables.

Foiling High-GL Carbs

You'll reduce the GL of a typical portion of any carb meal by combining in nearly any vegetable or fruit (again, potatoes do not count). If you include spinach, carrots, and tomatoes to a pasta salad, for example, you'll eat less pasta.

Should you add chopped broccoli into a rice side-dish, you'll eat less rice; the same goes for adding strawberries to warm or cold cereal. And fewer carbohydrates equal lower blood sugar.

Let us consider a rice side-dish. A portion of 180g of cooked long-grain white rice has a GL of 23, which makes it a high-GL food.

However, equal weight of boiled dried peas has a GL of only 3, so in the event that you mix an equal number of peas using the rice, a 150g portion of the side dish could have a GL of only 13, changing it from a high- to a medium- GL food.

Actually, combining any vegetable in your rice - chopped cooked onions or asparagus or carrots - likewise lowers its GL.

Snack Tips

Whole fruit is always a good snack option. For example, a 50g pack of potato crisps has a GL of 14 - making it a medium-GL food (but only when you consume this much with no more).

However, a medium peach or plum has a GL of only 5, and the GL of a similar sized apple is 6. Additionally, you are consuming twice as much food; therefore which do you think will probably fill your hunger best? The GL would be just 16, even if you ate a peach, a plum and an apple.

On the flip side, in case you munched your way through 100g of crisps, the GL for your snack would be considered a much bigger 28. Raw vegetables are also Super snacks, dipped in low fat sour cream, low-fat dressing.

Pack a few cherry tomatoes or carrot sticks in a sandwich bag and you'll not have any reason to hit the vending-machine. Fill up on veggies of various colors, since various colors indicate different health protective compounds.

Things Allowed

Just about all fresh garden produce is beneficial to us, but specific kinds are not as beneficial to our blood sugar levels.

When we mention to eat more veggies and fruits, we're referring to colorful vegetables (not starchy vegetables or potatoes) and fresh, whole fruit. A few examples below:

Potatoes

These really are the exception: they are dense in easily absorbed carbohydrates, so their GL is fairly high. Actually, the more potatoes, including chips, that an individual eat, the higher their threat of diabetes.

Many dietitians believe potatoes ought to be labeled with grains rather than with veggies, and even then they are at the peak of the carbohydrate pyramid.

Other Starchy Vegetable

Winter squash and sweet potatoes are rich in carotenoids and other essential nutrients as well as fiber, which can be advantageous. Although their carbs aren't readily absorbed as those in white potatoes, they are also high in carbs.

That makes a much better alternative to them than white potatoes, as with several other carbohydrate - rich foods, keep an eye on your portion size.

Juices

By drinking only the juice, you'll pass up on all the fiber and a few of the vitamins in the entire fruit, and also you'll get much more calories along with an increased GL.

If you eat 125g of fresh pineapple, for example, the GL is 6. But should you really drink a little glass (180ml) of pineapple juice, the GL is 12.

The same goes for grapefruit (GL 3) versus a little glass of grapefruit juice (GL 7), and for orange (GL 5) versus a little glass of juice (GL 10). Also if you go for a Hugh sweetened fruit drink, the GL soars: a 375ml glass of cranberry juice cocktail has a GL of 36.So if you drink juices, be attentive to keep portions small, and also make certain they are unsweetened (read labels carefully).

Dried Fruits

Drying concentrates the sugars in fruit and will make for intensely calorific treats. It is good to get some raisins, dried dates, plums, figs and apricots, but do not overindulge in them. Study what happens when plums (GL 5) turn into dehydrated prunes (GL 10) or grapes (GL 8) turn into raisins (GL 28). A handful, or 60g, of dried dates has a whopping GL of25.

Section 1- BEAUTY CARE

For several generations, the Japanese have recognized the benefits of vinegar as a beauty aid and, as Western consumers continue to seek skin friendly and natural treatments, vinegar sits in our cupboard as the achiever.

The styptic and toning qualities of vinegar, especially apple cider vinegar have for centuries been employed as part of women and men beauty regimes.

Vinegar is considerably more astringent than ice and will reduce redness, bruising, inflammation and swelling in about half the time.

Skin

Your Skin is damage by the environment, diet and the pressures of day-to-day life; therefore it deserves the very best care and treatment.

Vitamin C is an extremely important element for skin and, with the aid of vinegar; it is easily digested by the body.

Vinegar also helps to bring back the natural pH balance of the skin, so drink a teaspoon of apple cider vinegar in a glass of water each day.

Age Spots

Apply full strength apple cider vinegar dabbing with a cotton pad for about ten minutes two times per day to successfully repair your hands. The spots will fade in a couple of weeks. Age spots can be caused by hormonal changes, and due to over-exposure to the sun.

Dietary Changes Tips

Store all seeds and nuts in the refrigerator or freezer, as they can easily become rancid. Stay away from rancid oils. Refrigerate all oils; never store them on a shelf at room temperature once opened.

Grains should be stored in a cool, dry place. Stay away from all fried foods. Hot grease and cooking oils contain high amounts of skin-damaging substances.

Stay away from junk food, tobacco caffeine, alcohol, and sweets.

Cleanse your liver. Drink beet juice. Two or three ounces of beet juice per day will be sufficient in the beginning of your cleansing program.

As you detoxify your liver, you can increase your intake of beet juice to six ounces.

Nutrients That Helps

- Beta-carotene is an antioxidant that slows the aging process.

- Vitamin C is an antioxidant that helps in repairing tissue.

- Bioflavonoids work synergistically with vitamin C to repair tissues.

- Vitamin E is an antioxidant that reduces the aging process and helps repair tissue.

ACV Cosmetic Peel

The purpose of a cosmetic peel is to release the epidermis of the skin, eliminating a layer to expose the layer beneath. The hypothesis is the fact that the new skin encourages a fresher, younger-looking appearance but the procedure can be expensive.

This is also a gentle treatment, and if performed too harshly, faces can appear as if they can be gravely sunburned. A more affordable and simpler edition, which is often utilized for a home treatment, is the vinegar peel.

Scrub your face with your favorite scrub and then apply vinegar directly on your skin; leave for five full minutes. Rinse the vinegar off and your skin will feel soft and look much fresher. Your Skin will be sensitive to sunlight, so stay out of direct sunshine for an hour after treatment.

Broken Veins and Bruises

As a mild astringent, apple cider vinegar is a helpful treatment for all those miniature, but unsightly broken veins that may frequently appear on top of skin.

Dab on undiluted apple cider vinegar to reduce redness and speed up the repair once or twice a day. Bruises may also be treated in the same manner.

ACV Gets Rid Of Blackheads

Blackheads are annoying and embarrassing, the consequence of having a greasy skin or teenage acne. The property of strawberries when combined with vinegar provides a natural deep cleanser.

Combine 1/3 cup vinegar with five chopped strawberries and leave at room-temperature for a few hours. Strain the liquid through a sieve and remove the strawberry pulp.

Gentle, pat the liquid on to the area affected by blackheads before retiring to bed. Rinse off in the morning and repeat until the blackheads clear.

ACV Get Rid Of Acne

Acne is a general term often used to indicate acne vulgaris, which is a chronic inflammatory disease of the sebaceous glands and hair follicles of the skin. It is characterized by blackheads, whiteheads, and pimples. Chronic acne can result in scarring.

A contributing factor may be diet, as evidenced by studies of Eskimos and other cultures that first experienced acne after adopting the Western diet. Some acne is caused by a condition known as "skin hypoglycemia" or "skin diabetes."

This means that the skin (which is an organ) is intolerant to sugars. Acne can cause embarrassment and loss of self-esteem, and this is what every teenager's dread.

General References

Cleanse your face at least twice a day. After washing, apply benzoyl peroxide 5-percent gel at night. Extract blackheads every two or three days. Avoid using greasy creams and cosmetics, and avoid medications that contain bromides or iodides.

Dietary Changes

1. Eliminate sugars. A study has shown that skin glucose tolerance is significantly impaired in acne patients.

2. Eat a high fiber diet. Client's skin has cleared rapidly when fiber was increased in the diet. Foods high in fiber are fruits, vegetables, whole grain cereals, whole grain breads and crackers, bran, and legumes (beans, lentils, and split peas).

Nutrients That Helps

- Take Vitamin A to slow down the production of sebum. Be aware. Though, that Side effects may result from high doses of Supplemental Vitamin A. Beta-carotene, which can be

found in fresh vegetables and fruits, is a smarter choice. Beta-carotene is transformed into Vitamin A as your body needs.

- For acne breakouts, take Vitamin B6. It is helpful for premenstrual acne breakouts.

- Folic Acid can be helpful also.

- Selenium with vitamin E can regularize glutathione peroxidase levels.

- Chromium increases glucose tolerance levels and improves insulin sensitivity.

- For tissue regeneration and inflammation control, Zinc plays an important role in wound healing.

- A low-fat diet can be helpful along with essential fatty acids. A good source of omega-S fatty acids is pure cold-pressed flaxseed oil and cold-water fatty fish and green vegetables.

Acne Vinegar Remedy

A good remedy that is often used and is also economical and easy to make is a combination of one teaspoon vinegar to ten teaspoons water. Empty it into a little, handy bottle, through the entire day, dab it on to pimples and spots.

The skin will be helped by the vinegar mixture to get back to its normal pH balance. Another home treatment is to make a paste composed of two teaspoonful apple-cider vinegar, one teaspoonful of honey and one teaspoon of flour.

Leave this on overnight and rinse off in the morning. Always test it first on a single blemish; if it is effective, the blemish should heal quicker.

Prevent Flaking Skin and Oily Skin

Whether the skin is greasy or dry, apple cider vinegar is rich in acids that help to dissolve fat and reduce flaking while encouraging a softer, smoother complexion.

A combination of equal parts apple cider vinegar and water placed on the face, allowed to dry, then rinsed with water will enable your skin to breath much easier and look fresher.

A Radiant Glow

The cost of commercially skin treatments is sufficient to make you think that they work. However you can create your own natural treatments which will perform just as well.

Mix 1/2 cup olive oil with three teaspoons apple cider vinegar, diluted with enough water to create a cream. Apply small quantities to the face before bedtime and rinse off the following day with water. Your skin will feel moisturized and cleansed.

Tooth Care

Get rid of bad breath and whiten your teeth by brushing them a couple of times per week with white vinegar. Soak dentures overnight in warm water with 1/4 cup white vinegar. This will soften tartar so that it can be easily brushed away with a toothbrush.

ACV Aftershave

As an after-shave, small amounts of vinegar will keep the skin looking great and keep shaved skin disinfected. Use undiluted vinegar as an aftershave lotion, especially if commercial aftershaves cause itching and rashes. Your skin will be soft, and skin problems will be helped.

1. Tone facial skin using a solution of equal portions of vinegar as well as water.

2. Steam clean your face using apple cider vinegar.

3. Lean over a pot of boiling water (carefully at least 8-inches from the water) with a towel over your head to trap the steam. After a minute, apply apple cider vinegar

Get Rid of Dandruff

Vinegar has acetic acid, which destroys the Malassezia furfur (the fungus) and helps to repair the pH balance of the scalp. Start by using warm water to rinse your hair, and then apply a solution of apple cider vinegar to help facilitate the dandruff.

Try applying equal amount solution for an entire rinse, or treat a problem area by implementing a tablespoon of apple cider vinegar on the hair and massage gently with your fingertips, Wait a few minutes, then wash as normal and rinse well in warm water.

ACV Hair Conditioner

Whip together 3 egg whites, two tablespoons olive oil or almond and one teaspoon apple cider vinegar to bring the life back into limp or damaged hair with a nourishing hair conditioner.

After that, gently massage all the mixture into hair and then cover with a shower cap, leave on for thirty minutes. Rinse with warm water, shampoo and wash as ordinary.

Protect Your Blonde

Blonde hair needs additional protection, especially if you swim in chlorinated water. Rub apple cider vinegar in your hair and let it set for 15 minutes or so before you go for a swim.

Get Rid Of Head Lice

Dealing with head lice can be embarrassing. Washing hair with a solution of white vinegar helps to loosen nits from the hair shaft before applying a lice killing shampoo.

Apple Cider Vinegar Bath

There are various variations, starting with the basic process of adding 4 cups apple cider vinegar to the water. Herbs rose petals, chamomile. Adding vinegar to the water helps restore the pH balance of the skin.

While running the bath, scatter a handful of bruised mint leaves as well as one cup of apple cider vinegar in the hot water. Then leave the bathroom for a few minutes before climbing in the bath. The mint and vinegar will refresh and restore an aching body.

Chapping Nails

To stop your hands and nails from chapping and drying out, rub a little vinegar into them, they'll immediately soften.

Pedicure or manicure demands attention not just to the nails but to the cuticles too. Soften cuticles by soaking your toes and fingers in white vinegar for 5 minutes.

While you're pampering your feet take a second or two to inspect the state of your toenails. Wearing closed shoes for a long period where toes are in slightly damp and airless conditions can provide the ideal home for fungal infections.

Wrap feet in a washcloth dampened with undiluted vinegar, or soak feet in 1 part vinegar to 2 parts warm water. The vinegar will change the skin ph., stopping fungus growth as well as deodorized and softened feet.

Lasting Nail Polish

Your nail polish can lasts longer if the nails are dampened first with a cotton wool ball soaked in apple cider or white vinegar. Allow the nails to dry, afterward apply your favorite color.

Skin Toner

Dull skin tone makes the skin look older and uneven. Over exposure to sunlight, dietary intake, and aging can all contribute to dull skin tone. Apple cider vinegar is a good and effective remedy to brighten and tone your skin.

Apply apple cider vinegar to your face to get a smooth texture and appearance to the skin, control oil production and clear blemishes.

ACV is a natural antibiotic which also helps in reducing breakouts caused by bacteria and yeast. Apple cider vinegar also helps your skin to have more elasticity and keeps it youthful for longer.

Add equal parts of water and apple cider vinegar in a bottle. Add a few drops of your favorite oil and apply to your skin. Use as a daily toner.

Section 2 – HEALTH

Apple cider vinegar is the favorite curative vinegar and can be used in all of the treatments highlighted in this book. Natural apple-cider has more advantages; therefore as your own treatment base you can use it as often as you wish.

It has to be stressed that before self-diagnosis, it is essential to sit and talk to a medical practitioner about your health condition. The hints highlighted here are home cures only and each individual will have different answer to their complaint.

In most circumstances, just like any kind of drug or food, if the utilization of vinegar exacerbates your symptoms, discontinue treatment promptly and consult your physician.

Note!

Vinegar contains acetic acid, and acid and tooth enamel do not blend nicely. Bear in mind that as a treatment when ingesting vinegar, it's **RECOMMEND** to dilute it with water.

Prolonged utilization of neat vinegar can damage your teeth, to make sure you're on the safe side – dilute neat vinegar with water.

Prevent Stomach Problems

Apple cider vinegar contain a natural bacteria fighting power and contain potassium, chlorine, phosphorus, magnesium, sulfur, sodium, calcium, iron, copper and fluorine.

It has been claimed to relief individuals from heartburn, pain, indigestion issues, constipation, heartburn, and neutralize hazardous substance and bacteria.

Add one teaspoon of apple cider vinegar and one teaspoon honey to your juice or drink 30 minutes to one hour before your meal for the relief of indigestion, heartburn and nausea.

In addition, it can be added in soups, marinades, gravies, sauces, salads, and purees to add flavor. Pickles, relishes and chutneys prepared with apple cider vinegar can be made as part of each meal to add value to your diet plan.

Apple cider vinegar can be added during food preparation and can also be used in small amounts on a daily basis to enhance the peristaltic movements of the intestine. It is also proven to flush out toxic waste from the body which helps in keeping the digestive system in good condition.

Soothe Digestion Problems

ACV helps to boost the production of gastric juices and enzymes required for proper digestion when consuming food. These enzymes assist in the breaking down of foods into smaller bits so that the useful nutrients apple cider vinegar contains can be absorbed by the blood stream during digestion.

Consuming apple cider vinegar benefits the body by providing nutrition. It is also helpful in increasing the acidity of foods that's required for digestion. The presence of pectin which is a dietary fiber obtains a role in calming digestion and intestinal spasm.

Its antibiotic property can aid in relieving diarrhea caused by bacteria. The strong taste and smell of apple-cider vinegar can be difficult to consume at first, but after a few days it gets better, and becomes part of your daily diet.

Keep a bottle of ACV handy at all times in your kitchen to obtain the full benefits of the power of apple cider vinegar.

Soothe Sore Throats

Many sore throats are the result of bacteria or viruses invading the tissues lining the throat. A battle takes place between the invading army of germs and your body's immune system. The result of this battle is inflammation, which causes swelling and pain.

Your doctor may recommend antibiotics, which works by killing the bacteria. Over-the-counter drugs work by masking the symptoms.

The natural remedies below work by making your immune system stronger so that it can protect your cells from infection more effectively.

Some sore throats are caused not by infection, but by other irritants, including dust, smoke, fumes, extremely hot foods or drinks, or allergens such as pollen. Just like invading bacteria, these irritants cause the throat to be inflamed and painful.

Sore Throats Remedy

- Dip a fabric in a blend of 2 tablespoons of apple cider vinegar and 1 cup of warm water. Squeeze the fabric out and gentle lay it on your throat, to keep it from shifting from its place wrap another fabric around it.

Keep this on when going to bed. The power of the vinegar will pull all the toxins out of your body that causes the sore throats.

- In a cup of warm water, mix four teaspoons of honey and four teaspoons of apple cider vinegar. Drink every four hours.

- A 'raw throat' after a cough can be soothed by gargling with a mixture of 1 teaspoon salt and 1 tablespoon apple cider vinegar melted in a cup of mild warm water.

Use few times daily if needed. For sore throats associated with the flu and colds, blend equal amounts cider vinegar and honey, stir or shake until dissolved, take a tablespoon every four hours.

Common Cold

A cold is a viral infection of the upper-respiratory tract. It's very infectious, and incubation time is eighteen to forty-eight hours in length. Lasting immunity doesn't develop.

Cold symptoms include blockage of nasal passages using a watery discharge, sneezing, and headaches. A cold may also be accompanied by a dry sore throat, fever, body pains, fatigue, and chills.

Health Tips

The most powerful and effective method of preventing a common cold would be to strengthen the immune-system. More than one or two colds a year indicates weakened immunity. It's highly advisable to get checked for food allergies, if regular colds are experienced.

When you "catch" a cold, there are measures which you can take to shorten the recuperation time. Get lots of rest in bed. Jobs and other duties often push us to neglect the body.

But lack of rest can hinder the human body's defense mechanisms and extend infection. Especially when you sleep, and if you rest in bed, strong immune - strengthening substances are discharged, improving the potency of the immune functions. Drink lots of fluids.

Dietary Changes

- Beta-carotene supports immune function and heals the epithelial tissues that line the respiratory system.

- Vitamin C has antiviral and antibacterial action. This nutrient can shorten the length of the common cold, and it has proven valuable in prevention.

- Bioflavonoids act synergistically with vitamin C and have antibacterial actions too.

- Zinc has antiviral activity.

Common Cold Vinegar Remedy

One well known method of attacking a cold's development would begin with a warm bath. While in the bath, pour two cups of vinegar, get a washcloth, steep it inside the vinegar solution and put it on your own chest, keeping it in place for ten minutes. Rinse your chest. Repeat the process until the cold starts to leave the body's system.

For Your Health

Cholesterol is likely to stick like superglue to artery walls; Whereas Hyperglycemia creates unbalanced types of oxygen known as free radicals.

These horrible molecules harm the arteries, so it's tougher for the blood vessels to do their work of keeping your blood pressure stable. The amount of insulin the body demands to tame all this blood sugar is awful, too.

They can make blood more prone to form heart-threatening clots, set in place alterations that raise blood pressure, and increase swelling - all of which are demonstrated to increase your likelihood of cardiovascular disease.

The possibility of sudden cardiac arrest - and heart problems is expected to happen from food which cause blood sugar levels to rise are also prone to decrease 'good' HDL cholesterol and raise triglycerides, fats that are dangerous to cells.

Apple Cider Vinegar Benefits

Studies have shown how strong these treacherous effects can be for the heart. In a research of over 43, 0000 men aged 40 and older, folks whose diets intake increased the most to blood sugar were 37 percent inclined to experience heart problems in the following five to six years.

A recent health study of over 75,000 middle-aged American women, folks whose diets intake increased the most to blood sugar the most were two times as likely to experience cardiovascular disease over the next nine to ten years.

For obese women, this kind of diet was significantly more harmful. For example, their triglycerides were 144 per cent which is much higher than those women, who ate a healthy diet. Fortunately, the phenomenon works in contrary, also. The better your meals are for your blood sugar, the gentler they will be to your own heart.

Cholesterol Vinegar Remedy

Mix juices from fresh fruits which are also famous to aid in reducing cholesterol levels. Use fruits like, cranberries, apples and grapes. Add two tbsp. apple-cider vinegar and consume on a daily basis and watch as your cholesterol levels reduced.

Vinegar is acknowledged to lower cholesterol levels, because of its acidic nature found in vinegar as well as the rich mineral and trace element content assisting in bringing the body back to its normal equilibrium.

Clears Nasal Congestion

Apple cider vinegar helps in clearing nasal congestion by steam inhalation. You can add it to your humidifier for the best results or add the ACV to a bowl of hot water and inhale the steam from the ACV. The strong scent will relieves mucus from your nasal passage. Repeat two or three times daily.

Barbara B Walters

ACV For Hiccups

Hiccups normally last for a couple of minutes but at times can last longer. Hiccups are caused due to frequent contraction of diaphragm. Although folks mostly rely on home remedies such as drinking water or holding breath for hiccups, these remedies are slow in working.

A quick way to stop hiccups is to consume 1 teaspoon of apple cider vinegar and two teaspoons of honey in warm water. Apple cider vinegar facilitates proper contraction of diaphragm and stops hiccups within minutes.

Acid Reflux

Acids secretion helps with food digestion in the human stomach. Acid reflux occurs when the glands start secreting excessive amount of acids; irritation is caused by these acids in esophagus, causing nausea and stomach ache. With no side effects, apple cider vinegar is an effective remedy for this problem.

Reduce acids in apple cider vinegar reacts with strong stomach acids and corrects the pH balance in stomach. ACV does not only treat acid reflux but in addition it ensures appropriate functioning of the human stomach.

Acid Reflux Remedy:

Mix two table spoons of honey and white apple cider and drink before meals.

Arthritis

Arthritis is inflammation of the joint often accompanied by discomfort and, regularly, changes in structure. The most usual kinds of arthritis are rheumatoid arthritis and osteoarthritis.

Osteoarthritis

Osteoarthritis is a type of arthritis affecting the bones and joints. It's characterized by light early-morning stiffness, stiffness after lack of joint function, pain that's worse when the joint is used.

Symptoms can change from local tenderness, bony inflammation, swelling of soft tissues, and cracking of joints in motion to limited flexibility.

Osteoarthritis is separated into two groups primary and secondary. Primary osteoarthritis is a degenerative ailment as a result of deterioration on the body.

Secondary osteoarthritis is as a result of predisposing factors for example injury or prior to inflammatory disease of the joint.

Keep In Mind

Osteoarthritis sufferers should attain and keep normal body weight. Extra weight places an additional stress to the joints.

Dietary Changes

- Try taking away the aubergine, tomatoes, peppers, potatoes, and tobacco. Even if signs enhance a little continue to stay clear of these foods.

- Stay away from oranges, lemons, limes, and grapefruits. These are thought to result in joint swelling.

- Stay away from all refined meals for instance processed foods, white sugar and white flour as well as preserved foods.

- Eat a healthful diet focuses on vegetables, seeds, whole grains, (legumes split peas, lentils, and beans), fruits and nuts and includes a small part of low-fat animal products.

Nutrients That Help

- Methionine is significant in cartilage structures.

- Pantothenic acid can be useful, as a lack of this nutrient has been linked with osteoarthritis.

- Vitamin C may be helpful.

- Bioflavonoids have been proven to be helpful.

- Copper may possibly be useful, as a lack of the nutrient has been related with osteoarthritis.

Arthritis Vinegar Remedy

The process is simple. Begin by adding 1 tsp. of vinegar a day in a glass or cup of water. Over time, increase this to 2 times per day and drink with each meal.

At your very own speed, increase the vinegar intake to two teaspoon with each glass. Consult your doctor prior to starting any kind of treatment.

Insomnia

This section is about common sleeplessness not caused by discomfort or sickness. Drugs do not generally treat insomnia. They simply desensitize the mind for a while, often leaving a 'hang-over' next morning.

For many of us, though it occupies about one third of our entire lives, so we'd best learn how to-do it well. The effects of sleep are felt on the majority of our bodily functions.

The very first signal is a deepening of the respiration and a slowing of the heartbeat. The blood pressure falls. Your body temperature drops by about half a Fahrenheit degree (or even a quarter Centigrade).

The feet grow warmer and your hands colder. The sweat glands are active, so good ventilation is crucial. The blood supply to the brain will not decrease.

Apple Cider Vinegar Benefits

At this time, your brain is active during the night. The pupils of your eyes move quite fast, about one hour after you drift off. This movement appears as an important element of actually refreshing sleep and its onset and duration is delayed if sedative drugs are used.

What then can we learn from all this to help our slumbers? Firstly as evening approaches, you need to cultivate quite consciously a peaceful state of mind. Think about nice folks and great things.

Some mellow music often helps. It will be great if you have taken a little activity in the open-air - a short stroll, possibly, lively enough to tire you a little.

Remember that people need differing amounts of sleep although it is inconvenient in the event your partner needs twice (or half) as much as you do. When you grow older you are inclined to want less sleep.

It is good to really have a warm nourishing beverage half an - hour before retiring. Just before going to sleep drink cider vinegar and honey, 2 teaspoonful of each in warm water lie down, think pleasant thoughts and relax your body.

Diabetes

Diabetes results when the human body is no longer competent to correctly process blood glucose. A daily tonic of apple-cider vinegar can supply pectin, a water-soluble fiber good for helping regulate glucose levels.

Apple cider vinegar can additionally help restore digestion and nutrient absorption, since digestive functions have been impaired by many diabetes sufferers.

Urinary Tract

The goal of the urinary tract is to assist in removal of waste in your body and to do this it needs a certain number of acidity.

Coffee, antibiotics, infections and bacteria, each of these and many other phenomena can interfere with regular amounts of acid, making urination painful.

Vinegar's ability to repair pH levels will assist in restoring the tract to its normal state. Add 1 tsp. of vinegar to a glass or cup of water.

The Digestion

When you eat food it goes through a process of digestion in the mouth where the starches are turned, during the chewing process, into sugar by the enzymes in the saliva. It is important to chew thoroughly because chewing helps to break down the food and stimulate the flow of saliva.

The saliva is normally alkaline but the active enzyme works best in a slightly acid medium; therefore we have found our first indicator of the value of the cider vinegar drink in that it helps the upkeep of the desired acidity.

After the food has been formed into a conveniently sized portion you swallow it and it descends the eight or nine inches to the stomach which is a collecting sack for the food you eat.

The digestive process now carries on a further stage in the stomach. The gastric juices contain about 0.4 per cent of free hydrochloric acid together with enzymes which make the food liquid. Harmful bacteria and other organisms are usually made harmless whilst the food is in the stomach.

Digestion and absorption of the nutrients continues in the twenty- two feet long small intestine where there are more enzymes and a lot of valuable and essential bacteria which help to break down food into substances which can be absorbed by the body.

Indigestion Vinegar Remedy

Combine ½ a teaspoon of green tea extract and 2 teaspoons of vinegar and fill with boiling water in a small pot.

Allow the liquid to steep for 5 minutes then drink as needed. You can use peppermint tea instead; peppermint considerably helps digestion and is well known for its gains for dyspepsia (upset stomachs).

Dizziness

Dizziness can result from an alkaline condition in the body, as well as a number of conditions that affect the central nervous system by sending conflicting information from the eyes, ears, etc.

Many people find relief from dizziness by taking the apple cider vinegar tonic on a regular basis.

Ear Aches

Having an infection of the ear can be very painful. An effective and fast home remedy is apple cider vinegar. Rest the affected ear over a bowl of hot water, adding one part apple cider vinegar. Be careful not to hold your ear too close to the bowl. This provides relief from discomfort.

Allergies

Allergic rhinitis is the clinical term for your nasal symptoms due to allergies to airborne fragments. The illness can be an occasional irritation or a severe problem that affects each facet of daily life.

For thousands of individuals the simple act of stroking the cat or opening a window, produces sniffles and sneezes. The reason for the symptoms is an overactive immune system and not cat hair, dust or pollen.

If you have symptoms all the time - seasonal allergic reactions - the main possible root reasons are "pet" fur, mold and mildew or home allergen.

If you experience symptoms throughout warm weather you might have the seasonal allergies usually referred to as hay fever, stimulated by grass pollen or tree during late spring and early summer.

These irritants all create exactly the same symptoms. Individuals that suffer with allergic rhinitis frequently have a low level of resistance to sinus infections, flu, colds, and other respiratory ailments in some households, allergic rhinitis might be an inherited problem.

Causes

When germs, viruses or other substances enter the human body, the immune system attempts to destroy the ones that may cause disease or illness but ignores harmless particles including pollen.

In sensitive individuals the immune system cannot differentiate between harmful and benign material; therefore, innocuous fragments activate the release of the nature occurring substance called histamine and other inflammatory compounds within the area where the irritant entered the body - the nose, throat or eyes no one understands why the immune system overreacts in this way, but some specialists believe that poor diet and air pollution may weaken the system.

Remedy for Allergy Relief

It'll be really unpleasant on your throat, if you drink the apple cider vinegar direct. I advise drinking 1 - 5 teaspoon doses of unfiltered apple cider vinegar (raw) in a cup of mild warm water.

Raw, unheated honey likewise has anti-allergenic properties. You may include a small squeeze of lemon juice also. This is really a gentle method to consume apple cider vinegar."

Yeast Infection

One of the most reliable and natural remedies for curing yeast infection permanently is apple cider vinegar. ACV fights against harmful bacteria, while pharmaceutical medicines often kill good bacteria. External symptoms of yeast infection include burning of skin, itching, and rashes.

Apple cider vinegar can cure these symptoms. Pour 2-3 cups white apple cider vinegar to warm water and soak for 10 minutes. If the itching continues, repeat the process twice a day.

High Blood Pressure

High blood pressure is a common health problem; it often leads to nervous breakdown and stress. A number of people rely on prescribed drugs but most of these medicines lower blood pressure by controlling the nervous system.

These medicines are lifetime drugs and there are side effects of these medicines. However, using natural remedies for lowering high blood pressure can help in treating this problem without damaging your health. Apple cider vinegar is an effective and natural remedy for high blood pressure.

Apple cider vinegar acts as a health tonic by lowering the LDL levels and reducing the risk of diseases like high blood pressure. Apple cider vinegar is extremely rich in potassium. Add a mixture of 1 tablespoonful apple cider vinegar and 1 tablespoonful raw honey three times daily or before every meal.

Eczema

This condition has become synonymous with chronic dermatitis. In early stages, the skin may be itchy, red, and swollen, with small blisters and a weeping of fluids. Later, the skin generally becomes crusted, scaly, and thickened.

Other possible symptoms include burning, the appearance of papules, and a tendency for the skin to become overgrown with bacteria.

Studies have shown that eczema is, at least partially, an allergic response. Low stomach acid (hypochlorhydria) has been associated with both eczema and food allergies. Stress can also contribute to eczema.

General References

The control of food allergies is a very important part of eczema control. If you suspect that you are allergic to certain foods but are unsure as to which ones, ask your doctor for a food allergy screening test.

Skin-scratch tests are not always efficient means of determining food allergies; the RAST or ELISA blood test is recommended by many nutritionally oriented doctors.

Dietary Changes

- Increase your consumption of fatty cold water fish such as bluefish, herring, sardines, mackerel, salmon, tuna, Pacific oysters, European anchovies, and squid. People with eczema have shown a deficiency or defect in essential fatty acid metabolism. This defect appears to create a decreased formation of anti-inflammatory substances.

Studies have found that increasing the consumption of essential fatty acids by eating fatty fish at least twice weekly and supplementing with fish oils, flaxseed oil (expeller- or cold pressed), or evening primrose oil alleviates symptoms of eczema.

At the same time, the consumption of animal fats should be lowered, because these fats generate substances that are sources of inflammatory agents.

- Raise your consumption of oats, because they are found to have anti-inflammatory properties that are very helpful for eczema. Both raw and cooked oats are powerful. In Addition, an oatmeal facial pack may be beneficial.

(Mix one-half cup oats with water or a small yogurt, making a paste, and spread over face or other areas affected by eczema. Let dry for about fifteen minutes. Rinse well, and keep affected tissues clean and dry.) If there is any indication of infection, see your doctor. Do not attempt to treat infections yourself.

Eczema Vinegar Remedy

Eczema sufferers claim that using vinegar in their diet has significantly decreased and occasionally even totally eliminated their eczema.

Vinegar should have exactly the same effect on an eczema rash because it does on other types of skin irritation, when it is directly set on the affected region.

Pouring a tablespoon or 2 of cider vinegar in a bath can assist a lot also. Some eczema is an inner response to a reaction inside the body and in such cases vinegar might not help. Medical assistance should be sought, if this is the situation.

Skin Fungus

Apple cider vinegar is an effective health tonic it is a homogenous mixture of a number of acids and also an anti-septic solution. Apple cider vinegar can be used to treat all kinds of skin infections caused by fungus attack. Apply raw apple cider vinegar to the infected area. Repeat twice daily.

Psoriasis

This skin disease results when skin cells divide too quickly- up to 1,000 times faster than normal. The result is a pile-up of skin in the form of itchy silvery scales on the buttocks, scalp, and soles of the feet and on the backs of the wrists, elbows, knees, and ankles. In addition, toenails and fingernails may lose their luster and develop pits and ridges.

An outbreak can be triggered by stress, infection, illness, surgery, sunburn, viral or bacterial infections, or drugs like lithium. Psoriasis is most common between the ages of fifteen and twenty-five.

This disorder is not infectious, and presently there is no cure. Treatment consists of increasing compounds that cause skin cells to mature and decreasing compounds such as polyamines, which may increase cell overgrowth.

General References

Expose the affected area to sunlight for one hour each day. The application of heating pads has also proved to be effective. Both sunlight and heating pads may help to reduce the severity of symptoms.

Nutrients That Helps Psoriasis

- Zinc losses through skin shedding are greater in psoriasis. Zinc is also necessary for the absorption of linoleic acid, a fatty acid necessary for healthy skin. Pumpkin seeds are an excellent source of both zinc and linoleic acid.

- Selenium helps decrease the formation of inflammatory compounds.

- Folic acid may be deficient in psoriatic skin.

- Beta-carotene, which the body converts into vitamin A, decreases the polyamines, substances that are implicated in accelerating skin growth.

Psoriasis Vinegar Remedy

This skin condition is mostly treated by keeping the affected part (frequently the face and head) wet with swimming or bath. Oftentimes hot water can cause additional itchiness; therefore it really depends upon what works best for the person.

To alleviate an itching scalp, dip a fabric in apple cider vinegar and apply to the scalp or use a final rinse of vinegar in the water after washing your hair.

Memory

Iron helps transfer oxygen to the cells, and amino acids are crucial for the synthesis of brain chemicals; both of those factors help enhance memory. Apple cider vinegar helps the physical body metabolize iron and supply trace quantities of amino acids. Many experts believe that individuals using cider vinegar frequently in the diet have consistently great mental powers long into their old age.

Asthma

If you have had an experience of asthma, you're acquainted with the terrifying feeling of shorting of breathe "unable to breathe properly". Perhaps you are considering a home remedy to treat your asthma, despite the fact that you have an inhaler or drug.

Shake the vinegar well to mix the **"mother"** throughout the entire bottle. This has extreme healing properties; therefore it's essential to drink certain amount with each dosage. Add 1 tbsp. of the vinegar into a cup of water and mix it well. Drink it slowly in small sips for about an hour.

Repeat the same procedure after one hour, if wheezing has still not gone away significantly. Pour apple cider vinegar in a vessel or bowl and steep a cloth in, and then apply enough pressure as you hold it against the insides of your wrists.

Liver Function

For a good liver function. Add 1 tbsp. of apple-cider vinegar in your daily meal. This will assist in breaking down fats proteins as well as fats from the liver that can be trapped by rich foods.

Apple cider vinegar has always been considered a detoxing substance, so it is common sense that it would encourage the activities of one of our important toxin - removing organs, the liver.

Morning Sickness

The nausea of morning sickness can happen since the stomach has received no stimulation to create digestive acids following nights of inactivity, just as dyspepsia can become an issue of too little stomach acid, as opposed to too much. On occasion the most powerful remedy for not wanting to eat something is to eat just a bit.

Drinking apple cider vinegar tonic in small portions will help produce an appropriate balance of stomach acids. Occasionally nausea can be relieved by cooling the human body. Some experts advocate a compress put on the belly soaked in apple-cider vinegar.

Gallbladder – Gallstones

Apple cider vinegar may be used as part of a favorite alternative remedy referred to as a gallbladder flush. Likewise, straight olive oil is drunk at bedtime.

Olive oil is incorporate by some professionals with cider vinegar or apple juice, particularly for regular removal of small gallstones that are really not causing discomfort.

While painful gallstones ought to be treated by a doctor, a yearly gallbladder flush can help avoid the development of larger stones.

Hemorrhoids

The healing properties of full strength cider vinegar applied directly to hemorrhoids can cut back stinging and boost shrinking. Routine use of the cider vinegar can help soften stools and decrease the need for straining during elimination. This will definitely help prevent hemorrhoids in the future.

Section 3 – PETS

Vinegar plays a critical part in pet care, from keeping out unwanted pests such as ticks and fleas which can affect the health and well-being. Vinegar is also great for keeping pets living and sleeping areas clean and odor free.

❖ A neat way to remove water lines and deposits that form in fish bowls and fish tanks is to wipe them out with vinegar and followed by a rinse. Soak overnight for stubborn deposits.

❖ Treat animal (urine) stains on carpet as soon as possible. Blot up all liquid, and then flush the place a few times with plain water, blotting after each. The last step is to, flush with an identical parts water and vinegar. Rinse well and allow drying.

Pet Flea

ACV is an effective method that works fast to get rid of fleas. Having pets that's prone to fleas can be horrible! Add equal parts apple cider vinegar and water and give your pet a bath using a brush to gentle brush the hair.

Next, rinse the ACV mixture off your pet and dry. This will not only improve the coat of your pet but it will get rid of all the fleas. Your pet will thank you.

Pet Blankets

Wash your pet blankets as normal but add 1 cup white vinegar to the cycle to deodorize and kill bacteria when washing.

Your pets can have sensitive skin too. Use vinegar to remove any remains of soap from their bedding to which they are sensitive.

Cholesterol And Apple Cider Vinegar

Some level of cholesterol has to preserve the healthiness of the cells in the body and to also create hormones secretions that activate different organs and glands.

There are two kinds of Cholesterol, good cholesterol and bad cholesterol. Cholesterol is a waxy metabolite that exists in the blood HDL - high-density lipoprotein is called 'good cholesterol' and the human body is expected to increase the percentage of HDL in the body as much as possible. HDL helps eliminate the unwanted (poor) cholesterol from the walls of the blood vessels.

LDL-CHOLESTEROL or Low density lipoprotein is called 'unhealthy cholesterol'; it is responsible for making a soft, oily, wax-like plaque in the internal walls of the blood vessels.

Accretion of LDL in arteries can obstruct the vessels and may lead to inadequate stockpile of blood towards one's heart or brain. This problem can result in a heart-attack or even a stroke. Liver creates the required amount of cholesterol.

Apple cider vinegar helps the liver to maintain a regular flow of blood, and cleanse the body of toxins. For this reason, the vinegar will help to improve the function of the liver.

Blood Cholesterol Levels

Our physical body gets cholesterol from the food that we eat. In fact, cholesterol created by the liver is sufficient for the requirement of the body and we need not have it from outside. HDL needs to be above 60 mg/dL. HDL less than 40 mg/dL substantially increases the danger of cardiovascular disease as well as stroke.

LDL ought to be less than ONE HUNDRED mg/dL. LDL 130 - 159 mg/dL is considered as 'borderline high' and more than 190 mg/dL is taken into consideration as 'very high'. Overall cholesterol needs to be less than 200 mg/dL.

The ratio for ldl/hdl must be generally higher than 0.4; however any ratio above 0.3 is thought to be inside the usual levels of cholesterol range.

if you're thinking of trying apple cider vinegar for reducing the blood cholesterol , you could regulate this ratio, as it would allow you to understand if consuming vinegar has effectively worked for you or not. Reducing cholesterol levels without medication is possible, if you follow the information on reducing cholesterol.

Try to Include low fat dairy products in your diet on a daily base, eat good fats in the precise proportions, avoid high fat meat (have lean meat instead) and deep-fried foods. Staying clear of cholesterol rich meals such as egg yolk can assist in the prevention of high blood cholesterol.

Cholesterol Ratio and

Apple Cider Vinegar

Consuming Apple cider vinegar to reduce high cholesterol is an olden holistic treatment. Ayurveda doctors from ancient Egyptians and ancient India have announced endless benefits of the apple cider vinegar. They've used it habitually to treat sicknesses of all sorts, as they understood that it increased the flow of blood circulation to the body.

Most vinegar begins as fruit juice which is exposed first to yeasts, then bacteria, which work on fruit sugars in different ways. Initially these sugars are fermented by yeast to create alcohol.

Then specific bacteria break down the alcohol to form acetic acid, the main component in vinegar.

Both the yeasts and bacteria that make vinegar are plentiful in nature, so after the juices are extracted from the fruits, these liquids naturally progress through stages of fermentation, then acidification.

The vinegar dissolves mucous secretion, fat, cholesterol, arterial and joint deposits; that may cause serious health problems. Therefore, 'apple cider vinegar for high cholesterol' has become the essential phrase, when exploring the solutions to manage cholesterol.

By making dietary adjustments, it is possible to lessen as much as 30 percent of unnecessary cholesterol. Low cholesterol diet which includes foods that lower cholesterol normally is the best method to regulate blood cholesterol levels.

One tbsp. of Apple cider vinegar with a small amount of honey to add taste if taken every day, works great for blood cholesterol. You can use Apple cider vinegar instead of white vinegar when cooking, as it makes no distinction in taste.

Your cholesterol count will be within a healthful and protected range again. Vinegar also helps you to shed pounds naturally and alleviates joint pain.

Apple cider vinegar contributes to several roles when included in regular diet and helps improve your health and well-being in different ways.

Apple pectin, a water soluble dietary fiber existing within the apple-cider vinegar, consumes the fat molecules and unhealthy cholesterol. It boosts excretion of those unwanted substances and minimizes their levels. Liver plays an essential part within the metabolic processes, as you probably already know.

If the ingested food is not metabolized correctly, it contributes to 'weight gain'. Vinegar enhances the process of digestion of fatty meals. It can help speed up the metabolic rate of fats, proteins along with other elements present in food.

This way, it encourages weight loss. Therefore, health and wellness benefits of the Apple cider vinegar are of great importance. So, among each of the natural treatments, apple-cider vinegar is the number one choice.

Honey and Apple Cider Vinegar Benefits

A mixture prepared from honey and apple-cider vinegar has been utilized for an exceedingly long time to treat several illnesses, especially pain in the joint.

Even though this is actually the biggest perk of regularly drinking a glass of honey mixed with water and apple cider vinegar, you will find many other advantages of the two when consume on a regular base.

Whether on their own or together, apple cider vinegar and honey are beneficial for your body. On the next page, we have a look at apple cider vinegar and honey when mixed together and how it can be helpful to the body.

Benefits of Honey with

Apple Cider Vinegar

When taken together, honey and apple cider vinegar has great benefits to our health. Vinegar is a naturally acidic product, however, if consumed; it turns alkaline in the body.

The essence of the alkaline from the vinegar has made it an excellent treatment to respond to the ill-effects of a highly acidic diet that we eat in regards to fast food and so forth.

Furthermore, it is well-known to be used as an important treatment for pain in the joint and arthritis.

Honey gives a similar result when used as treatment as well. Though it has a reduced pH, it becomes alkaline as soon as it is consumed, and assists in the safe excretion of high levels of acids in the entire body.

Honey is normally added to apple-cider vinegar to ensure it is simple and easier to consume by toning down the sharp taste of the vinegar.

Even after that, you may not find the drink to be delicious. However, when you begin, you will want to keep consuming it on a regular basis, because of the adjustments you will start to experience within your body. A few of the perks you are likely to experience by drinking this mixture are given on the next page.

Benefits of Consuming

Honey and Vinegar

- Relief from indigestion or constipation
- Relief from joint pains
- Removal of halitosis (bad breath)
- Relief from sore throat
- Delayed aging process
- Reduced cholesterol levels and blood pressure
- Boosted stamina and energy levels
- Relief from pyrosis (heartburn)
- Weight loss

Apple Cider Vinegar

Health Benefits

- Apple cider vinegar helps with the treatment of sinus infection and clears sore throat.

- It helps in stabilizing the cholesterol levels.

- In regards to treating skin problems like acne, few come close the effectiveness of apple cider vinegar.

- Additionally, it shields us against most forms of gastrointestinal disorder.

- Apple cider vinegar assists in curbing allergic reactions in animals and humans.

- It reinforces our defense mechanisms and prevents muscle weakness after exercise.

- Vinegar raises the entire body's metabolism which encourages weight reduction, eliminates constipation and enhances digestion.

- A mix of lecithin and vitamin B6, and apple cider vinegar is thought to be among the best dietary medications for weight-loss.

- It relieves the pain from arthritis and gout.

- Its consumption prevents bladder stone and urinary tract infections.

- Vinegar has acidic properties, which is used for treatment for bad breath.

- The sulfur in apple cider vinegar helps to fights aging process. Thus, it's used as a treatment for liver spots.

- It is used by women as a treatment to reduced cellulite.

- It's also used for as a treatment for serious ailments such as hypertension and diabetes.

Honey Health Benefits

Honey is among the best treatments for arthritis. For treating arthritis, Combine and make a mixture of one teaspoon cinnamon powder, two parts lukewarm water and one part honey. Apply the mixture to the joints which is most distressing; this will lessen the pain in fifteen minutes.

Vinegar is also used for treating hair thinning and baldness. Before having a bath, prepare a mixture one tablespoon of honey, one tablespoon warm olive-oil, as well as a teaspoon of cinnamon powder, and apply the mixture on your scalp leave on for a few minutes.

Honey is also an effective treatment for toothache. Prepare a mixture containing five teaspoons of honey and one teaspoon of cinnamon powder, and apply it directly on the aching tooth.

Honey is quite effective, when it comes to lowering cholesterol. To lower cholesterol, make a combination of honey, cinnamon powder and 16 ounces of green tea. Drinking this mixture will lower the cholesterol level instantly.

It is quite powerful against acute coryza (common cold). Combine one tablespoon of honey with 1/4 tbsp. of cinnamon powder. Have this for three days; this will undoubtedly get rid of the cold. Honey combined with cinnamon powder also helps in reducing stomach ache.

For weight loss, prepare a concoction of honey with cinnamon powder and water, and consume it on a daily basis. This helps decrease the buildup of fats.

CONCLUSION

Whether your interest is in food that's both healthy and delicious, or in finding out if it works for you personally like a treatment, you cannot afford to be without vinegar.

Barbara B Walters

www.ingramcontent.com/pod-product-compliance
Lightning Source LLC
Chambersburg PA
CBHW060413290526
45791CB00002B/731